Tantric Alchemy
vs
The Doctors of Death

C. Lloyd Thompson

DEDICATION

To all of those who have faced the Beast

the fear mongers

and found some healing

without their permission

without a prescription.

CONTENTS

Acknowledgments   i

1   Believing   3

2   And the Doctors   Pg 7

3   Tantra   Pg 10

4   Alchemy   Pg 16

5   Awakening the Healer Within   Pg 22

6   Rise from your Deathbed   Pg 26

7   The Prize   Pg 28

8   Internal Alchemy   Pg 31

9   Chi Nei Tsang   Pg 37

ACKNOWLEDGMENTS

I am guided and protected in all things great and small.

Mother/Father God

Lord Shiva and Kalima be praised

BELIEVING

I started off believing and obeying like everybody else; feeling

paralyzed by the God-like powers of doctors. Like they have secret

knowledge to see into your soul and make a diagnosis of all your sins.

The verdict without a trial or hearing.

I got all caught up in the 60s drugs and revolution. Got locked up

like "One Flew Over the Cookoo's Nest". My street partner said,

"Run some shit on'em, get out of jail".

I got a diagnosis of Schizophrenic, paranoid type; transported to

the state mental hospital kind of like Ken Keasey in real life. I

thought it was kool being transported in chains, hand cuffed and the

waist in the back of a station wagon with an armed deputy sheriff

driving.

I meet another doctor/god in the nuthouse; askin funny questions

tryin to get me to reveal my inner knowledge, my secret spirituality so

they could prescribe a pill to kill it and give me shakes and tremors

3

instead.

The psychiatrist with deep dark circles around his eyes told me to stop writing poetry; like writing poetry was a contagious virus that led to mental illness. You do what they tell you because they have the power, wealth and keys and you hope to get out some day.

When I got out I was court ordered to a psychiatric social worker. He was teaching me how to take care of myself and take my pills. He took a shine to my hot, sexy wife. Not sure how that was supposed to work for my therapy and healing. Pretty sure neither one of them gave a rat fuck.

Then I was running wild on the road with a new sexpot wife. I was high all the time. Crashed and burned into a suicide ward in Bellingham Washington. Female shrink had an issue with angry men. 6'5" male nurse backing her all the time. Told me to baby-sit while my wife went on sex dates. She said, "It might be good therapy for you. Oh, and by the way, you're not schizophrenic. You're PTSD."

Later on;

Playin the game, going to college like that's what you do to cookies and live the dream. Thought I might as well try it out. Didn't have to take spinal tremor, brain damage, give you the shakes meds any more.

Now the doctors have Happy Pills. It's all about serotonin uptake. Let's call everything anxiety and depression now. "Get your happiness perscription."

Being in college makes you believe all the machinery might be built for you.

And

Your carnival ride is only a few good grades away. "Take your happiness pills and come get yours."

How many hours sitting in those intimate psychiatrist waiting rooms.

Peeking over the magazine, pretending to read.

Trying to guess, "What's wrong with her/him? They look sort of normal."

I look pretty normal too.

Nice new designer sneakers with all the technology power to walk to school.

AND THE DOCTORS

Those presiding Lords

only have 15 minutes

to assess meds and write a new script

and bless me with the hope of happiness

and sanity someday.

Somewhere there was a shift from psychiatry of lying on a couch and telling your dreams, fears and phobias to a relaxed foreigner with a notepad; going to unlock your inner soul to understanding and fulfillment. Was that only in the movies? Or just for wealthy people?

Or was it a shift in the working model with the discovery of magic pills to control symptoms and manipulate moods? The pharmaceutical giants began to influence medical schools, funding Doctors and research results that lay the groundwork to sell billions in drugs.

Insurance funded facilities only hire Doctors who subscribe to Brain-model psychiatry. Shamanic healing is demoted to dark-age superstition. Alternative herbal medicines are undermined with fear and the control thugs of the FDA. They enforce the drug dealer's territories just like gangs and crimes families.

Today there is some resurgence to the soul-body connection. Using ancient healing technologies to establish relationships between body-mind and biochemistry; the technology of miracles.

Diagnosis and treatment run hand and hand with mega-giant pharmaceutical companies that work hand in hand with international insurance companies that yield more political power with the ruling super powers than lesser nations.

I could feel their anti-depressants deep within my body....doing

something to my brain.....below the level of conscious decisions and

yet you can feel them doing what they know is best for my

biochemistry.....perhaps to make me more compliant to a military

complex?

I have done so many drugs that acutely affect brain function and

survived that I have mutated some inner-watching skills. This is what

the Shrinks call a non-compliant patient.

The drug was manufacturing an imbalance in the endocrine by

creating an artificial stimulation to provoke a burst of Serotonin into

the blood stream and flood the brain transmitters with this happiness.

It was nice to temporary relief from chronic depression. I didn't

know I was depressed because I had been pretty much constantly

depressed since childhood.

But....for some reason.....I didn't like the power of the pill taking

over my central nervous system and manufacturing moods. "Isn't it better to find the root causes and find natural means to stimulate the

glands into balance?"

TANTRA

Somehow I summoned the courage to face my own darkness. I decided to let go of anti-depressants as a way to cope with anything; pain, sadness, grief and general unhappiness.

I announced my intentions to the psychiatrist who was supervising me in 15-minute medication checks. He quoted to me grim statistics of suicide victims and those who end up locked in asylum wards as a result of refusing their pills.

Just to reinforce the fear tactics he had my final visit inside a locked psych ward with an armed deputy at the door. I could have been committed against my will. He did scare the shit out of me.

I felt like a condemned man walking on thin ice. I wonder if the pharmaceutical giants give doctors like him extra bonuses?

I didn't really have an alternative plan all worked out. At that time I didn't know of any alternatives. I just knew that something deep inside told me, "It's better to be dead than let yourself be an emotional puppet to a pill that takes over your brain.

My first self-treatment was to allow my depression to visit me. I didn't try to distract myself. I didn't try to find activities or substances to take my mind off the depression.

I said yes to all of myself. Whatever it is I want to embrace it, listen to it, get to know it like a friend I have been ignoring.

I had some horrendous personal losses at about the same time. Good reasons for anybody to pull their own plug; too much pain.

I had a full basement in my upper-Midwest home. I lived in a mostly black neighborhood of a major city. I didn't have much of a social presence. Nobody noticed the difference if I was in my basement alone pacing, howling, screaming. Or sitting alone at the top of the upper floor stairs; talking my madness out loud lost in my worlds with Ma Kali.

She never rejected my madness. It seemed like she used my madness to strip away more of my social conditioning and enter the fires of her pure, wild fierceness.

She accepted the sacrifice of my social conditioning and helped me go deeper into my wildness. Taboo worship of a goddess that my neighbors considered evil.

My depression wasn't healed and removed. It lost its meaning. Instead of removing it to make me presentable and socially acceptable Kali helped me to go deeper into my madness and wildness.

Dancing in the fires of the fierce forms of Kalima depression lost its meaning. I dwelled with adoration of her necklace of shrunken human skull and her mini-skirt of severed human hands.

My mental illness and social dysfunction faded. I performed sex acts with a deity nobody could see. Most said she was the queen of demons; or just my hallucinations.

When I first entered 12-step recovery from alcohol and drug addiction I had hit rock bottom. I was mentally gone from numbing out depression and anxiety with drugs and alcohol most of my life.

Spiritually I hit bottom. All my religious affiliations had left me bankrupt. I tried most versions of Christianity and only got tied in knots; probably psychotic from the their ideas of what it all means. Growing up in a predominantly Christian culture, it's either that or damned to Hell and torment.

They say, "When the student is ready, the teacher appears." I hit enough of a bottom to become willing to let go of old ideas and try something new. I was already damned by the Christian religion so I didn't have too much to loose there.

ALCHEMY

I opened up and began to experiment with other religious philosophies and practices. I spent a lot of time in nature, camping, hiking and being alone; away from the evils of society.

I was on my last Mountain Man run in N. W. Montana when I began my recovery. It was Old School, primitive living; chopping wood, carrying water, living without electricity or indoor plumbing. Doing everything by muscle and will power.....I blew my back out. I heard the pop of the ruptured disc.

Spirit has ways of forcing us to let go of old thinking and ways of doing things. I was very strong and tough with a high tolerance for pain. I could push myself beyond fatigue. "Push harder and ignore the pain." was my internal mantra.

I had to be cripples before I put up the flag and surrendered. They took an MRI of my back and gave me the news. 5 lower vertebrae degenerated with bulging disc, extreme sciatica, and extreme pain shooting down my leg. I also had a congenital birth defect in lower spine with curvature causing a slight twist. That may have been the weakness that led to all the injuries. Chronic back pain from doing back breaking work much of my life.

They wanted to cut bone off my hip to fuse together my lower 5 vertebrae. They also wanted me to begin taking Opiate pain pills. I couldn't sleep and I blacked out from pain rushes when I stood up.

I had another version of the depression dilemma. The doctors and specialists all agreed that I had to do it their way or I was doomed. I talked to many back surgery survivors while I was taking my physical therapy. None of them healed or recovered. Almost all of them ended up having three surgeries, chronic pain, disability, accelerated aging and a life long addiction to Opiates.

That's when I met my first Chinese Martial Arts teacher. Francis taught Tai Chi in a local Science of Mind church. I told him of my dilemma. "I think we can help you. But it will take time and lots of patience.

I began showing up at the weekly Tai Chi classes. But, since I was so severely injured, he gave me a few simple exercises to do while the class moved and flowed with grace and agility.

I didn't know it at the time. That was my first introduction to Chi Kung. Other fully functional students came and went. Sometimes I was the only one who showed up for class. So, I got a personal introduction to internal martial arts.

Francis encouraged me to travel and visit as many styles and practice centers as I could. I met many teachers of various skill levels. I experienced different styles and traditions.

I still felt like a fractured piece of China. I was very afraid of physical sparring as it could destroy me into 100 pieces and end my life. I never forgot what it was like to be crippled and helpless.

After about 16 years of Tai Chi; Yang style, Sun style and Chen Style I began to heal. In those days we didn't use the term Chi Kung. It was part of our martial arts warm up routines before we began forms work or paired practice.

I saw a posting for a Kung Fu class at a midwestern university I was attending. Something in me felt bold enough to risk it. I thought my sense of frailty might be safe in a university class setting.

It was Wing Chung Kung Fu from the lineage of Master Cheun. Demonstrating fighting application in two-person practice was a regular aspect. I had 16 years of Zen-based Karate and 16 more years of Tai Chi; Yang, Sun and Chen styles. I had never done actual sparring.

When we paired off to practice a technique or move I thought, "This is easy." I could see a number of weaknesses in the footwork, which could be exploited. The techniques were OK. But they were riddled with assumptions I was trained to not allow; or atleast not easily.

So, I played with my practice partners. I denied the move and or provided a lethal counter move. I knew Tai Chi was supposed to be the ultimate fighting art. I didn't know it was literal.

The Sifu intervened and asked me to let them do the move so the class could learn. I was sort of marked in the class as a showoff who knew other styles.

Sticky hands is the Wing Chung way of learning to feel, stick and follow. It's the essence of close-quarters fighting systems. The Sifu chose me as his practice partner. He's the one who sits on the panels that determine black belt degree.

I wasn't trying to do anything. I was playing the game. I thought everything was going fine. The Sifu got really upset because he lost my hand and had to look down to see that I was still in contact with him. He looked at me like, "No more magic tricks. Let's try that again."

AWAKENING THE HEALER WITHIN

Something happens when you practice internal martial arts for many years. It is called different names. In my Chi Kung system I call it Shen. It is the energy of emptiness. Not the emptiness of negative desolation. It is the emptiness of pure potentiality. We sort of experience it by accident when we are not really trying; just relaxed and letting things flow.

When I went in for my annual physical exam the doctor told me I has an elevated white blood cell count; probably because you have been sick. "Still, why don't you come in and get blood work again."

I will always remember the smugness on the doctor's face when he told me I had a form of Leukemia. It seemed that he loved the power of mutated diseases that took people down who have been health conscious. "Try to get out of this one Mr. Healthy Living."

He looked very happy as he explained, "There is no treatment, no known cure. It slowly progresses until it explodes in grizzly expressions." And then to add a cheerful note, "But, if you have to have something, this is the stuff to have because it is slow moving."

I felt paralyzed and very very alone. I already dealt with high blood pressure. It's a miracle I didn't have a stroke or heart attack from the sheer weight of it. That was the other tid bit of optimism he gave me, "Something else will probably take you out first.....like heart failure."

It seemed like there should be some super-hero that comes in to grab these inhuman care providers and give'em what they got comin. Instead they all cash in hundreds of thousands on each victim of modern disease. Everybody gets a share, a boat, a car, and a plane....something expensive.

And the bodies pile up and they make money off that too.

I tend to be hardheaded. I've been down for the count so many times I lost count. People and situations celebrating my demise because I was certain to not survive....whatever it was.

"You better make sure they're dead before you count Coup."

I rarely do what I am told to do. So, I began using my research skills. I don't take no for an answer unless it's the answer I'm looking for.

Many of the herbs with healing properties also had aphrodisiac profiles. They treat some sort of sexual dysfunction and contribute to healing major illnesses in males and females.

I spent several thousands of dollars in the first few years of research and experimentation. Fortunately for me, my disease was a slow moving one. The best I got in the early going was to possibly slow it a little bit more.

I had not found my answer yet. Like a mystic scientist, I had countless short-term results only to have them fizzle long term. I could still feel the lymph nodes swollen in my throat.

The doctor referred my to a cancer specialist. He did a bone

marrow extraction for laboratory analysis; DNA sequencing, state of

the art diagnostic technology. It is better than the terror of

wondering. "When will it go off? When will I be one of those

shuffling cancer-skeletons?"

RISE UP FROM YOUR DEATHBED

My neck felt hot to the touch. I knew I was laying on my deathbed. I kept researching; mostly because it is doing something other than just waiting to die.

I found a Chi Kung meditation called Microcosmic Orbit Circulation. I began getting up out of my deathbed to practice that. Later on I found the Bone Marrow Cleanse meditation.

I was willing to try anything if it had a possibility of working. I found and began to practice 8 Pieces of Brocade; the 6 Healing Sounds and began to practice.

I was still managing high blood pressure with pharmaceuticals. So, I had a yearly check up exam. I warned the practitioner that I would have a high white blood cell count because of the cancer that I live with. He gave me a blank look like, "Are we talking about the same thing here?" The white blood cell count was normal.

Traditional Chinese medicine is referred to as 5-element medicine. Taoist medicinal and martial arts refers to the 12 meridians associated with the 5 elements; 6 Yin and 6 Yang.

Medicinal Chi Kung continually refers to 5-element practices and balancing of the 12 meridians either directly or indirectly through traditional Chi Kung practices:

8 Pieces of Brocade, sitting and standing

6 Healing Sounds

5-element dance

5-element tapping and chanting

Bone Marrow Cleanse meditation

THE PRIZE

Taoism has religious goals. I refer to my practice as Tantric Taoism.

We look at the religious goals of various religions:

Christianity seeks to save your soul from a sinful nature

Buddhism seeks to enlighten the individual by awakening their

Buddha nature

and thus end the cycles of birth, death and more Karmic birth

Tantra seeks Moksha, absolute liberation

freedom from the slavery of duality and illusion

Taoism seeks to birth an immortal fetus within the adult body

long life and then immortality

We keep all this in mind when we enter the realm of Chi Kung

meditation. This has similarities with all meditation practices. Quiet

the mind. Let go of distractions and go deeper.

I call Chi Kung spiritual technology. The lower tan tien is about two finger widths below the navel. It is the element of water; Jing Chi which is the regenerative essence of life, sexual energies, the lower reservoir. It is closely related to the Kidneys and Bladder, which are the Yin and Yang meridians of the element of water.

In medicinal Chi Kung we seek to cultivate Jing Chi in the lower reservoir. When the lower reservoir fills with Jing Chi it begins to overflow into the 8 vessels. The vessels are connected to the meridians. The meridians are connected to vital organs.

When the overflowing reservoir begins to flood the vessels it is like irrigation ditches. The vessels are the large irrigation ditches that catch the runoff of the overflowing reservoir. When the vessels become flooded they feed the meridians. When the meridians are flowing in balance and rhythm we achieve rejuvenated health and long life.

The middle tan tien is called the heart center. It is the heart-fire.

This is called Yang Chi. it is located a little above the solar plexus.

The upper tan tien is called Shen. It is the energy of sacred emptiness; all-knowing, pure potentiality. It is located between the eyebrows and up just a little.

INTERNAL ALCHEMY

I usually like to introduce students to Internal Alchemy mediation of Chi Kung. Students with no experience seem to pick it up instantaneously.

I love sitting cross-legged on the floor for Zen meditation. But for Chi Kung meditation I recommend sitting on a chair with feet on the floor without shoes. Sit up straight. Don't lean back against anything. Feet planted firmly on the floor in a relaxed manner.

Begin by finding the breath. Just listen to your breathing to find where it is. Is it high in the chest? Is it shallow or strained? Relax the breath down to the belly. Begin natural belly breathing. The belly expands on the in-breath. The belly contracts on the out-breath.

Just relax into that for a few moments. Listen and feel your breathing. Let the breath become smooth and even. The lower tan tien is being massaged. The Jing Chi is being moved like gentle waves in the lower reservoir. The sexual, regenerative energies are being activated.

Now let your attention drift up to the middle tan tien just above the solar plexus. This is the Heart-fire of consciousness. The Witness-mind pays attention to the process. The Monkey-mind is at rest. We don't need to figure anything out. We don't try and make it happen. We witness and behold the effortless unfolding.

And so we become aware of a space between the Heart-fire and the Jing-chi. It is a space recessed back, a little towards the Kidneys. This is the space of the inner cauldron.

We visualize the water of the Jing-chi rising to fill the cauldron while we continue our rhythmic belly breathing.

As the cauldron is filling we visualize the heart-fire Chi sinking down until it is directly below the cauldron, which is filled up with Jing-chi. Each breath is like a billows tending the heart-fire as it heats and cooks the Jing-chi.

We notice that a vapor begins to form on the surface of the cooking waters of life. This vapor is called the Elixir of life.

The Elixir naturally rises up to the upper tan tien, which is between the eyebrows.

The Shen receives the Elixir and automatically becomes an open portal. The Elixir naturally flows into the open portal of the upper tan tien. It flows directly into the brain to nourish. The brain soaks up the Elixir like a sponge.

We continue the belly-breath like a steady bellows for the heart-fire cooking the regenerative sexual energies of Jing-chi. The Elixir continues to rise as vapor off the caldron.

The witness-mind looks to the crease between the hemispheres of the brain. This is called Spirit Valley. When the brain has become saturated with Elixir. The vapor drifts down the Spirit Valley to the back of the brain. This is directly below the Crown Chakra.

The Crown Chakra automatically opens when the Elixir reaches it. The Crown Chakra is in line with a straight spine. A beam of pure energy flows into the opened Crown Chakra. The Elixir naturally flows with the pure energy of the higher beings down the spinal column.

These higher beings are known by different names: spirit guides, teachers, masters or the spiritual language of any religion. I think of them as Shinning Ones, Star People, transcended immortals; the hierarchy of evolved beings up to the original beings, Mother/Father God.

Instead of praying with our thoughts, we are downloading directly. Their pure energy comes down through the spinal column mixed with the Elixir. It flows down and around the tailbone and back into the reservoir of Jing-chi to replenish and revitalize.

This is often where people meet their teachers and guides with direct experience.

We continue our bellows breathing, our circulating of Elixir for a few orbits until the Witness Mind focuses on the upper tan tien,

Shen. We notice with the Witness-mind that a second beam of pure energy radiates out from the Shen (third eye) portal.

This beam transcends the space/time continuum dimension. In the reality of this beam there is no relative time/space. All time is now; past, present and future.

In this pure beam of energy there is no distance. All space is here and now. We are free to travel and witness and receive visits.

We are connected through the Crown Chakra to the pure divine energy streaming down the spine. We are also emanating a pure beam out through the third eye.

If we are sitting in a meditation circle we now say our silent requests for the help and healing of situations and people. We also become willing to be used as channels to fulfill requests that we do not need to know the specifics of.

And then....there is a point of saturation. We begin to pull back to just the belly breath. The heart-fire returns to the center tan tien. The cauldron withdraws back to its enclave. Our portals naturally close. We come into our normal consciousness in the circle with others who are also coming back from super-here and now to the ordinary here and now.

CHI NEI TSANG

The abdominal area is the focus for many ailments. In Chi Kung we frequently twist the spine and waist. This squeezes and massages the intestines and internal organs.

This helps to dislodge gas bubbles, which are called Sick Winds. Some even refer to them as Evil Winds. They are sometimes released as belches, farts and various breathing noises.

So, in conclusion of our Internal Alchemy practice we begin to do some hand movements like Cloudy Hands holding the Energy Ball. As we pass this ball across the abdomen we also turn the waist and massage the intestines, stomach and organs.

We begin with the right hand on top of the ball, breathing rhythmically with belly breaths. After a few breaths you feel it natural to begin turning the energy ball each pass across the abdomen.

After a few breaths we naturally feel we are ready for release of Sick

Winds with a hissing breath through the teeth as you pass the energy ball across the abdomen. And then it becomes more of a vibrating OOOOO. And then on the next pass it becomes HAAAW with the hissing breath.

Follow the order of sounds until it is time to be still; breathing and doing nothing, listening. Sometimes it is helpful to place the palms face up on the knees; forming an energy triangle with the opened Shen/third eye.

When it feels natural come back into the room; rubbing the palms together, stretching and looking.

It is often useful to finish the practice with a talking circle. People share as they are comfortable about their inner experiences.

Bow and close; sometimes with hot tea and social time.

ABOUT THE AUTHOR

It's been 20 years since the Cobra bite

Kali

Her Kundalini serpent has fully risen now

I'm weaving together the threads

www.ingramcontent.com/pod-product-compliance
Lightning Source LLC
Chambersburg PA
CBHW071152220526
45468CB00003B/1024